The Fertility Diet Reset

A Guide to Preconception Nutrition and Awareness

Virgie W. Miller

COPYRIGHT

TABLE OF CONTENTS

CHAPTER 4

THE PLAN FOR FERTILITY DIET

INTRODUCTION

A Vital Component of Fertility: Diet

Our dietary decisions, in particular, have a significant impact on the process of conception. Fertility is greatly influenced by nutrition, which serves as the cornerstone for reproductive health. Fertility can be improved in both men and women by choosing the correct nutrients, which is more important than merely eating healthily. The important relationship between nutrition and the body's capacity for reproduction is examined in this section.

Essential Elements for Healthy Reproduction

Folic Acid: Neural tube defects are prevented and DNA synthesized.

Iron: Essential for encouraging ovulation and preventing anemia.

Omega-3 Fatty Acids: Essential for controlling menstrual cycles and producing hormones.

Calcium: Essential for promoting embryonic growth and preserving a healthy pregnancy.

Vitamin D: Essential for absorbing calcium and associated with better reproductive results.

The Reset Fertility Diet Method

Starting a family is made easier with the Fertility Diet Reset, which is a whole preconception nutrition plan rather than just a diet. It's intended to reset your body by feeding it foods high in nutrients that increase fertility. This strategy is a customized plan that takes into consideration each person's unique dietary demands and preferences rather than a one-size-fits-all approach.

Tailored Dietary Programs

Assessment: Analyzing eating patterns and nutritional conditions.

Customization: adjusting the diet to achieve particular reproductive objectives.

Implementation: Making the diet a part of regular activities.

The Fertility Diet Reset seeks to facilitate conception by emphasizing nutrient-dense foods and avoiding those that can impair reproductive processes. This proactive approach to improving fertility is backed by clinical experience and scientific study.

We'll go into greater detail about the Fertility Diet Reset as the book goes along, giving you the information and resources you need to make wise choices for your preconception diet.

CHAPTER 1

A GUIDE TO FERTILITY

The Fertility Biology

The ability to bear children naturally is called fertility. It is an essential component of human biology and involves intricate mechanisms controlled by both sexes' reproductive systems.

Regarding Women: The Menstrual Cycle

Menstruation: The uterine lining sheds.

An egg is released from the ovaries during **ovulation.**

Fertilization: The process by which an egg and sperm combine to create a zygote.

Implantation refers to the zygote's insertion into the uterine wall.

Sperm Production for Men

Spermatogenesis: The testes' process of producing sperm.

Ejaculation: The urethra is used to discharge sperm.

Variables Impacting Fertility

Fertility can be affected by a wide range of factors, including biological and lifestyle-related ones.

Factors Related to Biology

Age: As people age, their fertility naturally decreases, especially in women over 35.

Genetic Disorders: Reproductive health may be impacted by specific genetic diseases.

Hormonal imbalances: May cause problems for men and women during sperm production and ovulation.

Lifestyle Factors

Diet and Nutrition: Hormone levels and reproductive function can be impacted by inadequate diet.

Weight: Hormone production and fertility can be impacted by being overweight or underweight.

Substance Abuse: Use of alcohol, tobacco, and other drugs can have a deleterious effect on fertility.

The Effects of Nutrition on Reproductive Health

Our fertility can be significantly impacted by the stuff we eat. The quality of eggs and sperm, hormonal balance, and general reproductive health are all influenced by the nutrients we eat.

Foods That Encourage Fertility

Vitamins and Minerals: Reproductive processes are supported by vitamins and minerals including zinc, D, and folic acid.

Healthy Fats: The synthesis of hormones depends on omega-3 fatty acids.

Proteins: Offer the building blocks necessary for tissue growth and repair.

Fertility Dietary Patterns

The **Mediterranean diet**, which is high in fruits, vegetables, whole grains, and seafood, has been linked to improved fertility.

Plant-Based Diets: These may be advantageous provided they contain all the essential nutrients.

The foundation for comprehending the complex interplay between nutrition, lifestyle, and fertility is laid forth in this chapter. It emphasizes how crucial nutrition is to preserving reproductive health and fostering an environment that is conducive to conception.

CHAPTER 2

THE BASIS OF NUTRITION FOR FERTILITY

The Function of Macronutrients in Fertility

The main energy sources necessary for all bodily functions, including the reproductive system, are macronutrients.

Energy Source: Carbohydrates supply the energy needed for the metabolic processes involved in reproduction.

Fiber: Consuming a diet high in fruits, vegetables, and whole grains can help control insulin and blood sugar levels, which is important for maintaining hormonal balance.

Proteins: Growth of Cells: Proteins are essential for the development of reproductive cells as well as for the growth and repair of cells.

Sources: It's good for fertility to include both plant-based proteins (such as beans and lentils) and lean animal proteins (like fish and fowl).

.

Fats

Hormone manufacturing: The manufacturing of hormones requires healthy fats. They are important for both ovulation and the menstrual cycle.

Types of Fats: To promote reproductive health, a focus on monounsaturated and polyunsaturated fats, like those in avocados, almonds, and seeds.

Fertility and Micronutrients

Micronutrients are essential for fertility and should be ingested in sufficient proportions, even if they are needed in lesser amounts.

Vitamin D: Linked to improved reproductive outcomes, vitamin D supports endocrine system function.

B vitamins: They are necessary for DNA synthesis and the prevention of birth abnormalities, especially folate.

Minerals

Iron: Better ovulatory function is linked to an appropriate intake of iron.

Zinc: Needed for healthy egg and sperm production as well as cell division.

Phytonutrients and Antioxidants: Protectors of Reproductive Health

Phytonutrients and antioxidants guard the body's cells—including the reproductive cells—from harm.

Vitamin C and E are antioxidants that shield the body's cells from oxidative stress, which can have a deleterious effect on fertility.

Selenium: An antioxidant that helps shield chromosomes from harm.

The phytonutrients

Fruits and vegetables include flavonoids, which have been demonstrated to enhance sperm quality.

Carotenoids: They may increase fertility and are good for general health.

People can improve their fertility by making educated dietary decisions by knowing the significance of macronutrients, micronutrients, antioxidants, and phytonutrients. This chapter advises on how to incorporate each vitamin category into a diet that supports fertility as well as a thorough analysis of how each one affects reproductive health.

CHAPTER 3

FERTILITY-SUPPORTING FOODS

Superfood for getting started

Incorporating specific nutrient-rich foods might be especially helpful when making pregnancy plans.

Berries and Seeds

Antioxidants found in blueberries and raspberries shield reproductive cells.

High in **omega-3 fatty acids**, which are essential for hormone balance, are chia and flax seeds.

Zinc, which is essential for cell division and the development of healthy eggs and sperm, is abundant in pumpkin seeds.

Almonds: Offer a good amount of vitamin E, which can improve sperm and egg quality.

Produce and Fruits

Citrus Fruits: Vitamin C, which is abundant in oranges and grapefruits, helps enhance the absorption of iron and balance hormones.

Dark Leafy Greens: Rich in folate, iron, and calcium, these vegetables are great for a healthy pregnancy. Examples of these are spinach, Swiss chard, and kale.

Complete Grains

Quinoa and Brown Rice: These grains are great providers of fiber and complex carbs, which enhance ovulatory activity and help control blood sugar levels.

Leafy Greens and Nuts

Kale and spinach are great providers of folate, which is necessary to avoid birth abnormalities.

Walnuts and almonds: Offer vitamin E and good lipids that promote cell health.

Foods High in Protein

Beans and lentils: Rich in protein and fiber, they help maintain hormonal equilibrium.

Salmon and Sardines: High in vitamin D and omega-3 fatty acids, which are crucial for fertility.

Eggs: Have choline, which is necessary for the development of the fetal brain.

Lean Meats: Iron and protein are found in chicken and turkey, but they don't have extra fat.

Foods to Limit or Steer Clear of

Several foods and drugs should be avoided because they may negatively impact fertility.

Expensive Fish

King Mackerel, Swordfish, and Shark: High mercury concentrations in these fish may hurt reproductive health.

Soy-Based Products

Processed Soy: Although soy has some health benefits, it's best to avoid processed soy products because they frequently include additives.

Refined Sugars and Carbohydrates

White bread and pastries: These can raise insulin and blood sugar levels, upsetting the balance of hormones.

Sugars and Processed Meals

HIgh-Sugar Snacks: This may cause insulin resistance, which may interfere with ovulation.

Processed Meats: Frequently made with chemicals that could interfere with hormone function.

Alcohol and Caffeine: Excessive use of tea and coffee may be related to problems with conception.

Alcoholic Beverages: May have a deleterious effect on menstrual periods and sperm quality.

Decisions: Organic vs. Non-Organic

The argument over whether eating non-organic or organic food matters when it comes to preconception nutrition.

Fertility and Pesticides: Organic produce is grown without the use of synthetic pesticides, which can disrupt the balance of hormones.

Non-Organic Risks: These may include residues that are hazardous to the health of the reproductive system.

The Price and Availability

Cost-effective Solutions: Invest in organic foods for goods with a high pesticide risk and non-organic foods for things with a low risk.

Local and Seasonal: Getting organic food may be less expensive if you select locally grown and in-season vegetables.

The Advantages of Ethnic Foods

Decreased Chemical Exposure: Growing organic food can reduce chemical exposure because it doesn't require artificial fertilizers or pesticides, which is beneficial for general health.

Environmental Impact: Organic agricultural methods are intended to be less damaging to the environment and more sustainable.

Making Knowledgeable Decisions

The Dirty Dozen is a list of produce items that usually have high levels of pesticide residues. Selecting organic varieties of these foods can help lower your exposure to dangerous chemicals.

On the other hand, produce on **The Clean Fifteen** is typically free of pesticide residues, which makes non-organic selections more tolerable.

People can make dietary decisions that help their journey toward fertility by concentrating on superfoods, being aware of foods to avoid, and thinking about the organic versus non-organic issue.

CHAPTER 4

THE PLAN FOR FERTILITY DIET

Meal Planning Strategy for Optimal Fertility

A well-planned diet can have a big impact on fertility. It guarantees that you take in enough amount of the nutrients required to maintain reproductive health in a balanced manner.

Structure of Daily Meals

Breakfast: To balance blood sugar levels, start with a high-protein meal.

For **lunch**, prioritize a substantial ratio of nutritious grains, lean protein, and vegetables.

Dinner: More veggies and a lower protein intake are the main features, just as lunch.

Snacks: To sustain energy levels, have two snacks—one in the afternoon and one in the middle of the morning—that are made of fruits, almonds, or yogurt.

This is an example of a diet designed to promote optimal fertility:

Day 1

Breakfast consists of an omelet with spinach and mushrooms, whole grain bread with avocado, and mixed berries.

Mid-afternoon snack: Greek yogurt topped with almonds and seeds

Lunch consists of steamed broccoli and quinoa salad with grilled chicken.

Snack in the afternoon: hummus-topped carrot sticks

Dinner is Quinoa pilaf and Baked Salmon with Roasted Sweet Potatoes and Asparagus.

Evening Snack: Almond butter on sliced apples

Day 2

Smoothie made with berries, spinach, and chia seeds for **breakfast**; whole grain English toast with almond butter

Mid-morning snack: cottage cheese topped with pieces of pineapple

Lunch would be a whole grain roll and lentil and vegetable soup.

Granola and Greek yogurt for a **midday snack**

Dinner is mixed beans and vegetables with turkey chili.

Mixed greens, avocado, and tomatoes in a side salad

Snack in the evening: Greek yogurt with almonds and honey

Day 3

Breakfast consists of mixed fruit salad and avocado toast with poached eggs.

Mid-morning snack: cucumber slices and hummus

Lunch consists of brown rice, stir-fried veggies, and chickpeas, and steamed edamame.

Snack in the afternoon: guacamole and bell pepper slices

Dinner is grilled zucchini and bell peppers filled with quinoa with a side salad.

Snack in the evening: cottage cheese and peach slices

Day 4

Breakfast consists of whole grain muffins, Greek yogurt parfait, and mixed berries with granola.

Mid-morning snack: apple slices with almond butter

Lunch consists of a whole grain roll, spinach salad, and grilled shrimp with balsamic vinaigrette.

Trail mix with almonds, seeds, and dried fruit for an **afternoon snack**

Dinner is roasted chicken with lemon and herbs, quinoa, and roasted veggies. There's also steamed spinach on the side.

Mango coconut chia pudding for an **evening snack**

Day 5

Breakfast consists of scrambled eggs with spinach and feta cheese; whole grain pancakes with fresh blueberries and a honey drizzle.

Greek yogurt with sliced banana and a dash of cinnamon for a **mid-morning snack**

Lunch consists of grilled salmon salad, quinoa tabbouleh, and mixed greens with avocado and citrus vinaigrette.

Afternoon Snack: Almond butter on celery sticks

Dinner is brown rice, stir-fried vegetables, and steamed broccoli.

Snack in the evening: cottage cheese with slices of pineapple

Day 6

Breakfast consists of whole grain toast with mashed avocado and cherry tomatoes or chia seed pudding with mixed berries and sliced almonds.

Trail mix with almonds, seeds, and dried fruit for a **mid-morning snack**

Lunch consists of roasted sweet potatoes, lentils, and kale salad, and whole grain rolls with tahini dressing.

Greek yogurt with honey and walnuts for an **afternoon snack**

Dinner is baked chicken with quinoa crust, butternut squash, and roasted Brussels sprouts. There's also a mixed green salad dressed with balsamic vinaigrette.

Evening Snack: Almond butter on sliced apples

Day 7

Breakfast consists of a whole-grain English muffin with almond butter and a green smoothie made with spinach, kale, pineapple, banana, and coconut water.

Mid-morning snack: slices of peach and cottage cheese

Lunch would be a salad of chickpeas, avocado, cherry tomatoes, and cilantro-lime dressing. Grain-based pita bread

Snack in the afternoon: hummus-topped carrot sticks

Dinner is quinoa, roasted asparagus, and baked cod with lemon and herbs. Steamed green beans are provided.

Greek yogurt topped with a mixture of fruit and honey for an **evening snack**

A range of nutrient-dense foods are included in these meal plans to promote healthy eating and maximum fertility. Adapt meal selections and portion proportions to suit dietary requirements and personal tastes. Have fun while eating!

Preconception Recipes

Feta and Spinach Omelet

Ingredients:

- two eggs
- 1/4 cup crumbled feta cheese
- 1 cup fresh spinach - 1 tablespoon olive oil
- To taste, add salt and pepper.

Guidelines

- In a pan over medium heat, warm the olive oil.
- Transfer the beaten eggs into the pan from a bowl.
- Place feta cheese and spinach on top of the eggs.
- Fold the omelet in half after cooking until the eggs are set.

- Accompany with a piece of whole-grain bread.

Quinoa and Black Bean Salad

Ingredients

- One cup of quinoa; two cups of water
- one can of black beans, drained and rinsed
- one diced red bell pepper
- quarter cup chopped fresh cilantro
- Two tablespoons of lime juice
- One tablespoon of olive oil
- To taste, add salt and pepper.

Guidelines

- After rinsing with cold water, drain the quinoa.

- Boil the water, add the quinoa, lower the heat, cover, and simmer for fifteen minutes.
- Once the quinoa has cooled, fluff it with a fork.
- Combine the quinoa, black beans, cilantro, and bell pepper in a big bowl.
- Combine the olive oil, lime juice, salt, and pepper in a whisk and drizzle it over the salad.
- Before serving, toss to mix and chill for at least half an hour.

Broccoli and Almond Soup

Ingredients

- One tablespoon of olive oil
- one sliced onion
- two minced garlic cloves
- Four cups of florets of broccoli

- Four cups of vegetable broth; half a cup of chopped and roasted almonds
- To taste, add salt and pepper.

Instructions

- Heat the olive oil in a big pot over medium heat. Cook the onion and garlic until they become translucent.
- Add the vegetable broth and broccoli. When broccoli is tender, reduce heat and simmer after bringing to a boil.
- Use an immersion blender or a standard blender in batches to puree the soup until it's smooth.
- After adding the roasted almonds and returning the soup to the pot, season with salt and pepper. Serve warm after thoroughly heating.

Lentil Salad with Roasted Vegetables

Ingredients

- One cup of green lentils
- two cups of water
- One sliced zucchini
- One chopped red pepper, one chopped yellow pepper, and one tablespoon of olive oil
- Half a tsp balsamic vinegar
- To taste, add salt and pepper.
- Chopped fresh parsley (for garnish)

Guidelines

- Set oven temperature to 400°F, or 200°C.
- After rinsing, place the lentils in a pot with water. After bringing to a boil, lower the heat and simmer for 20 minutes or until the food is soft.

- Add a little olive oil, salt, and pepper to the bell peppers and zucchini. Arrange onto a baking sheet and bake for approximately 20 minutes, or until soft and beginning to turn golden.
- After draining, put the lentils and the roasted veggies in a big bowl.
- Add a balsamic vinegar drizzle and toss to coat. Before serving, garnish with fresh parsley.

Spinach and avocado smoothie

Ingredients

- One ripe avocado, scooped and pitted
- Two cups of raw spinach
- One banana
- half a cup of Greek yogurt
- One cup of almond milk
- One spoonful of honey, if desired

Instructions

- Blend all ingredients.
- Process till smooth. Add extra almond milk to the smoothie if it's too thick to get the right consistency.
- If you want your smoothie sweeter, taste it and add more honey. Serve right away.

Smoothie to Boost Fertility

Ingredients

- One ripe banana; half a cup of frozen berries (strawberries, blueberries, or raspberries); and one cup of spinach
- Half a cup of Greek yogurt
- One-third cup of chia seeds
- One tablespoon (optional) of maple syrup or honey
- One cup of almond milk, or any other type of milk.

Guidelines

- Place spinach in a blender along with frozen berries, banana, Greek yogurt, chia seeds, and honey or maple syrup (if desired).
- Cover the ingredients with almond milk.
- Blend until creamy and smooth.

4. Transfer into glasses and savor right now.

Kale and Quinoa Salad

Ingredients

- 1 cup cooked quinoa
- 1 cup chopped cherry tomatoes
- 1 diced cucumber
- 1/4 cup finely chopped red onion
- 1/4 cup pitted and sliced Kalamata olives
- 1/4 cup of feta cheese, crumbled
- One tablespoon lemon juice - Two tablespoons extra virgin olive oil
- One teaspoon of oregano, dried

- To taste, add salt and pepper.

Guidelines

- Put the cooked quinoa, cherry tomatoes, cucumber, red onion, olives, and feta cheese in a big mixing bowl.
- In a small bowl, mix together the olive oil, lemon juice, dried oregano, salt, and pepper to make the dressing.
- Drizzle the quinoa salad with the dressing and mix thoroughly.
- You can serve cold or room temperature.

Salmon baked in a pan with roasted veggies

Ingredients

- Two filets of salmon - Two tablespoons of olive oil - Two minced garlic cloves
- 2 cups chopped mixed veggies (carrots, broccoli, and bell peppers)

- 1 teaspoon dried dill

- 1 teaspoon lemon zest

- Salt and pepper to taste

Guidelines

- Preheat the oven to 400°F, or 200°C.

- Arrange the salmon filets on a parchment paper-lined baking pan.

- Combine the olive oil, dried dill, lemon zest, minced garlic, salt, and pepper in a small bowl.

- Coat the salmon filets with the olive oil mixture.

- Toss the mixed veggies with any leftover mixture of olive oil.

- On the baking sheet, arrange the vegetables around the salmon.

- Bake for 12 to 15 minutes, or until the veggies are soft and the salmon is cooked through, in a preheated oven.

- If preferred, serve hot with quinoa or brown rice on the side.

Salad with Avocado and Chickpeas

Ingredients

- 1 diced ripe avocado
- 1 can washed and drained chickpeas
- 1 cup halved cherry tomatoes
- 1/4 cup finely chopped red onion
- 2 tablespoons chopped fresh parsley
- 2 tablespoons lemon juice
- Two tsp extra virgin olive oil
- To taste, add salt and pepper.

Guidelines

- Combine the chopped avocado, chickpeas, cherry tomatoes, red onion, and fresh parsley in a large mixing dish.

- In a separate bowl, mix the lemon juice, olive oil, salt, and pepper to make the dressing.
- Drizzle the salad components with the dressing and toss to fully incorporate.
- Serve cold as a wholesome and revitalizing salad.

Soup with Lentils and Veggies

Ingredients

- 1 cup rinsed and dried green lentils
- 4 cups vegetable broth
- 2 chopped carrots
- 2 chopped celery stalks
- One chopped onion
- Two minced garlic cloves
- One teaspoon each of ground cumin and turmeric
- salt and pepper to taste
- optional garnish of fresh parsley

Guidelines

- Put the dried lentils, carrots, celery, onion, garlic, cumin, turmeric, salt, and pepper in a big pot.
- Bring ingredients to a boil over medium-high heat.
- Once the lentils and vegetables are soft, reduce the heat to low, cover, and simmer for 25 to 30 minutes.
- Taste and, if necessary, adjust seasoning.
- Spoon soup into dishes, top with sprigs of fresh parsley, if using, and serve warm.

Spinach and Berry Salad with Lemon Dressing

Ingredients

- 1 cup mixed berries (strawberries, blueberries, and raspberries)
- 4 cups baby spinach leaves
- 1/4 cup of almonds, sliced
- Two tablespoons of crumbled feta cheese (optional)
- Two tsp orange juice
- One tablespoon of juiced lemon
- One tablespoon each of extra virgin olive oil and honey

Guidelines:

- Toss baby spinach leaves, mixed berries, sliced almonds, and crumbled feta cheese (if using) in a large salad bowl.

- To make the dressing, combine the orange juice, lemon juice, honey, and olive oil in a small basin.
- Pour the salad with the dressing and toss to fully coat.
- Serve right away as a wholesome and revitalizing salad alternative.

Stuffed Bell Peppers with Quinoa

Components

- Four large bell peppers, any hue
- One cup of washed quinoa
- 1 can of rinsed and drained black beans - 2 cups vegetable broth
- One cup of corn kernels, either fresh or frozen
- Diced tomatoes, one cup
- One teaspoon each of chili powder and ground cumin
- To taste, add salt and pepper

- Optional: add 1/2 cup of shredded cheese

Guiidelines

- Set the oven temperature to 190°C, or 375°F.
- Slice off the bell peppers' tops, then take out the seeds and membranes.
- Combine the quinoa and vegetable broth in a medium-sized saucepan. After bringing to a boil, lower the heat to a simmer, cover, and let the quinoa cook for approximately fifteen minutes, or until the liquid has been absorbed.
- Put the cooked quinoa, black beans, corn, chopped tomatoes, cumin, chili powder, salt, and pepper in a big mixing basin.

- Place the filled bell peppers upright in a baking tray after stuffing them with the quinoa mixture.
- Top the stuffed bell peppers with cheese, if using.
- Bake the baking dish in the preheated oven for 25 to 30 minutes, or until the bell peppers are soft, covered with aluminum foil.
- Take out of the oven, then serve warm.

Buddha Bowl with Sweet Potato and Chickpeas

Ingredients

- 1 can of rinsed and drained chickpeas
- 2 tablespoons olive oil
- 1 teaspoon each of ground cumin and paprika
- 2 medium sweet potatoes, peeled and cubed

- 4 cups mixed greens (such as spinach or kale) - Salt and pepper to taste
- 1/4 cup tahini
- 2 tablespoons lemon juice
- 1 sliced avocado
- Two tsp water

Guidelines

- Set the oven's temperature to 400°F, or 200°C.
- Toss sweet potatoes and chickpeas in a big bowl with olive oil, paprika, cumin, salt, and pepper until well-covered.
- Arrange the chickpeas and sweet potatoes in a single layer on a parchment paper-lined baking sheet.
- Roast for 25 to 30 minutes in a preheated oven, or until the chickpeas are crispy and the sweet potatoes are soft.

- Make the tahini dressing by blending tahini, lemon juice, and water until smooth, while the chickpeas and sweet potatoes are roasting.
- To construct the Buddha bowls, divide the mixed greens among serving bowls, then add the avocado slices, chickpeas, roasted sweet potatoes, and tahini sauce on top.
- Present right away and savor!

Coconut Mango Chia Pudding

Components

- One-quarter cup chia seeds
- One cup of coconut milk
- One mature mango, chopped and skinned
- One tablespoon of optional maple syrup or honey
- Optional shredded coconut as a garnish

Guidelines

- Place the coconut milk and chia seeds in a mixing dish. Mix thoroughly to blend.
- Once the chia pudding has thickened, cover the bowl and place it in the refrigerator for at least 4 hours or overnight.
- Puree the chopped mango in a food processor or blender until smooth. Sweeten with maple syrup or honey, if preferred.
- To assemble, arrange mango puree and chia pudding in serving jars or glasses.
- If preferred, garnish with shredded coconut.
- Serve cold as a tasty and nutrient-dense snack or dessert.

Portion Quantities and Timings

Keeping a diet that promotes fertility requires knowledge of serving amounts and eating schedules.

Serving Size Guidelines
- 2 to 3 cups of **vegetables**
- 1.5 to 2 cups of **fruits**
- 6 to 8 ounces of grains, at least half of which should be whole grains;
- **Proteins**: 5 to 6.5 ounces daily
- **Dairy**: 3 cups daily for foods high in calcium

Consumption Pattern
Meals: There are three main meals a day, which are evenly spaced out between breakfast, lunch, and dinner.

Snacks: Eat two snacks to control hunger and avoid extended periods between meals.

These dishes are meant to be high in nutrients, offering a range of vitamins and minerals that are crucial for good health before conception. They contain foods like legumes, nuts, and leafy greens, which are rich in iron, folate, and other nutrients that promote fertility. Remember that throughout the preconception stage, a varied, well-balanced diet is essential. Savor these meals while you work toward a safe and healthy pregnancy!

CHAPTER 5

ADDING EXTRAS TO YOUR DIET FOR FERTILITY

Vital Add-ons for Getting Ready to Procreate

A balanced diet is the foundation of good health, but to make sure you're getting all the nutrients you need during the preconception stage, several supplements can be helpful.

The role of **folic acid** is critical for both avoiding neural tube abnormalities and DNA synthesis.

Dosage: 400 micrograms (0.4 milligrams) per day is the recommended amount by the US Public Health Service.

Iron's role in preventing anemia and promoting oxygen transport is crucial for ovulation.

Dosage: varies according to personal requirements; see a medical professional.

The generation and control of hormones depend on **omega-3 fatty acids**.

Sources: Algae-based products or fish oil supplements for vegans.

Vitamin D's role includes being essential for calcium absorption and is associated with better reproductive results.

Dosage: It's recommended to get levels evaluated and adjust supplements based on the amount, as this can fluctuate.

Acetaminophenol

Role: The antioxidant properties of this amino acid may enhance sperm motility and promote fertility.

Pyridoxine, or vitamin B6, is essential for the development and healthy operation of red blood cells as well as the synthesis of energy. Elevations of B6 in the blood have been linked to higher rates of conception.

Zinc: Zinc is necessary for DNA synthesis, cell division, and cellular function. Healthy growth and development are also dependent on it, from conception to adulthood.

Function of **Coenzyme Q10** (CoQ10): Serves as an antioxidant and may enhance the quality and maturation of eggs.

The purpose of **selenium** is as an antioxidant that helps shield chromosomes from damage and is crucial for thyroid health, both of which have an impact on fertility.

Myo-Inositol Role: May enhance ovulation and is frequently used to treat PCOS, a prominent cause of infertility.

L-arginine Function: This has been connected to enhanced sperm production and may enhance circulation to reproductive organs.

Melatonin's role: well-known for controlling sleep, this hormone also contains antioxidants and may enhance the quality of eggs.

Comprehending Supplement Labels

To make sure the supplements you're taking are appropriate for your needs, it's important to read their labels carefully.

Important information about serving size and servings per container is how much of the supplement is suggested daily and how long a container will last.

Use of Percent Daily Value (%DV): Ascertains how much or how little a supplement adds to your daily intake of nutrients.

The purpose of the ingredients list is to list all of the supplement's active and inactive ingredients, as well as any possible allergies.

Advantages and Dangers of Typical Supplements

Although there may be health benefits to supplements, there are also hazards to consider.

Advantages

Nutrient Deficiency: Iron deficiency, for example, can be prevented or treated with the aid of supplements.

Health issues: Vitamin B3 is one supplement that helps lower the risk of some health issues, such as hypertension.

Dangers

Overuse: Excessive supplementation can have negative effects like toxicity or drug interactions.

Quality Issues: Not all supplements are made equal; some might not have the specified concentration of nutrients or might contain impurities.

It's crucial to speak with a healthcare professional before taking any supplements for preconceptions to customize the dosage to your specific needs and guarantee safety. This chapter offers a thorough review of the main supplements that can help with fertility, as well as information on how to read supplement labels and weigh the advantages and disadvantages of popular supplements.

CHAPTER 6

ENVIRONMENTAL AND LIFESTYLE FACTORS

The Effects of Exercise on Fertility

An important part of a healthy lifestyle is frequent physical activity, which can also improve fertility.

Benefits of Moderate Exercise:

A Balancing Act: Moderate exercise can balance hormones, boost blood flow to the reproductive organs, and enhance general health.

Intensity: While strenuous activities could be advantageous, an excessive amount of high-intensity exercise may interfere with menstrual cycles and lower fertility.

Low-impact workouts are great for enhancing general health and have special advantages for fertility.

The following list of suggested low-impact activities can help to promote fertility:

Yoga: Increases blood flow to the reproductive organs, lowers stress levels, and increases flexibility.

Walking: Develops endurance and is a mild form of exercise that doesn't put too much strain on the body.

Mild Bike Rides: These can be a soothing form of exercise and have cardiovascular advantages.

Swimming: This exercise is great for individuals attempting to conceive because it works the entire body and is gentle on the joints.

Tai Chi: A mind-body exercise that lowers stress and encourages relaxation, both of which are good for conception.

Toxins in the Environment and Fertility

The fertility of both men and women can be negatively impacted by exposure to specific environmental pollutants.

Plasticizers are common toxins to stay away from because they include chemicals that can interfere with endocrine function.- Pesticides: Reduced sperm quality and ovulatory problems have been related to exposure to specific pesticides.[8].

Limiting Exposure

Food and Water: To reduce your exposure to dangerous chemicals, use glass or stainless steel containers instead of plastic ones.-
Household and Garden: Adopt natural pest management techniques and refrain from storing food in plastic containers.[8].

Techniques for Stress Management

Stress management is essential for preserving general health and has a favorable impact on fertility.

Practical Methods

Relaxation Techniques: Methods like yoga, meditation, and deep breathing help lower stress levels and enhance the success of conception.[11].

Time in Nature: Being outside helps reduce stress hormones and promote mental clarity.

Daily Integration - Routine: To manage stress proactively, incorporate stress-relieving activities into your daily schedule.

Support System: To provide emotional support, and keep a solid support system of friends and family.

People can establish an environment that is favorable for conception by making educated decisions about the effects of environmental pollutants, stress, and exercise. The data presented here is based on recent studies and our understanding of the contributions of these variables to fertility. Always remember that before making big lifestyle changes, especially ones that affect fertility and preconception health, it's advisable to speak with medical professionals.

CHAPTER 7

EXTRA ATTENTION TO DETAIL

Endometriosis and Polycystic Ovary Syndrome (PCOS)

For those who are impacted by PCOS and endometriosis, it is essential to comprehend how these disorders affect fertility.

PCOS: Fertility and Hormonal Imbalances

Features: Polycystic ovaries, increased testosterone levels, and irregular menstrual cycles are characteristics of PCOS.

Impact on Fertility: PCOS-related hormone abnormalities can cause ovulatory dysfunction, which makes conception difficult.

Pelvic Pain and Reproductive Health in Endometriosis

Overview of the Condition: Endometriosis is characterized by the formation of tissue that resembles uterine tissue outside the uterus, which can lead to pain and infertility.

Fertility Issues: Because endometriosis can impair the quality of eggs and implantation, between 30 and 50 percent of women who have the illness may have infertility.

Diet and Fertility in Men

Male fertility is significantly impacted by diet, which also affects the quantity and quality of sperm.

Nutrition's Effect on the Health of Sperm

Antioxidants: Vegetables and fruits high in antioxidants help shield sperm from harm.

Omega-3 Fatty Acids: Found in fish and nuts, these fats are vital to the integrity of the sperm membrane.

Age-Related Problems in Fertility

Age-related decreases in fertility impact both men's and women's chances of conception.

Female Fertility Decline

Quantity and Quality of Eggs: As women age, their eggs become fewer in number and of lower quality.

Menopause: Usually occurring in the early 50s, menopause prevents natural conception.

Changes in Male Fertility

Aging can lower sperm count and quality, which can impact an egg's capacity to fertilize.

Testosterone Levels: As people age, their testosterone levels may decline, which may result in decreased sperm production and erectile dysfunction.

This chapter discusses the unique factors that need to be taken into account while managing PCOS-related, endometriosis-related, male-specific dietary impacts, and age-related reproductive problems. To successfully traverse these issues, it is crucial for people and couples to be aware of these concerns and to seek advice from healthcare specialists.

CHAPTER 8

TRACKING YOUR DEVELOPMENT

Monitoring Your Dietary Consumption

Fertility depends on eating a balanced diet, and keeping track of your nutritional consumption will help you make sure you're getting the correct kinds of nutrients.

Techniques for Monitoring

Food Diaries: Make a daily log of all the food and beverages you consume.

Nutrition Apps: Make use of apps that can monitor and calculate your calorie consumption and macronutrient intake.

Signs of Fertility and What They Indicate

Understanding your body's cycle and recognizing your most fertile days can be accomplished by recognizing fertility markers.

Important Indicators of Fertility

Basal Body Temperature: A small increase in body temperature may be a sign of ovulation.

Cervical Mucus: Variations in the material and hue can indicate when fertility is expected.

Making Use of Ovulation Forecasting Kits

LH Surge Detection: The spike in luteinizing hormone that occurs before ovulation can be identified with ovulation prediction kits.

When to Get Expert Assistance

To properly handle fertility concerns, knowing when to seek help can be essential.

Rules for Requesting Assistance

Under 35: Seek assistance following a year of unsuccessful infertility attempts.

Over 35: Seek assistance following six months of unsuccessful attempts.

Irregular Cycles: It's best to see a specialist if your menstrual cycles are irregular or nonexistent.

Expert Assessment

First Assessment: To find any underlying problems, a healthcare professional might carry out a preliminary assessment.

Specialist Referral: For more thorough testing and treatment choices, you might be sent to a fertility specialist if necessary.

Understanding fertility indications and keeping track of your progress through nutritional tracking can provide you with valuable information about your reproductive health. Knowing when to get expert assistance when problems develop can result in prompt and effective interventions.

CONCLUSION

It's time to consider the information and realizations obtained as we draw to a close with "The Fertility Diet Reset." This journey has involved more than simply food; it has been a whole strategy for improving fertility through conscientious eating and lifestyle decisions.

A Summary of the Fertility Path We've looked at the science of fertility and learned how diet has a direct impact on reproductive health.

- We've found nutrients and superfoods that can help you in your journey to becoming pregnant.
- We've learned the value of meal preparation and come across meals that feed both the body and the spirit.

- We've explored the world of supplements, knowing when and how to select the right ones for our needs.
- We've talked about how stress, the environment, and physical activity affect fertility.
- We've discussed the special considerations for endometriosis and PCOS, as well as the effect that age and male fertility play.
- We've now covered the significance of tracking development and knowing when to seek expert advice.

Keep in mind that every step you take toward becoming pregnant is a step closer to your objective. Your daily decisions, ranging from what you eat to how you handle stress, all contribute to your overall health and well-being.

Keep Learning and Changing Your Diet and Lifestyle to Support Your Fertility Journey: Remain Hopeful and Informed Maintain contact with medical experts who can offer assistance and direction.

Accept perseverance and patience. Recognize that every reproductive journey is different and may require some time. Appreciate the little triumphs and persevere with fortitude and hope.

Your experience with "The Fertility Diet Reset" demonstrates your dedication to laying the greatest possible groundwork for pregnancy. With what you've learned and the habits you've created, you're in a good position to keep making decisions that will benefit your general health and fertility. Cheers to your triumph and the thrilling voyage that lies ahead!